MEDICAL HEALTH CLINIC
A Social Care Guide

MEDICAL HEALTH CLINIC
A Social Care Guide

LEON LOWE

Copyright © 2016 by Leon Lowe.

ISBN:	Softcover	978-1-5144-6487-8
	eBook	978-1-5144-6486-1

All rights reserved. No part of this book may be reproduced or transmitted in any form or by any means, electronic or mechanical, including photocopying, recording, or by any information storage and retrieval system, without permission in writing from the copyright owner.

Any people depicted in stock imagery provided by Thinkstock are models, and such images are being used for illustrative purposes only.
Certain stock imagery © Thinkstock.

Print information available on the last page.

Rev. date: 02/09/2016

To order additional copies of this book, contact:
Xlibris
800-056-3182
www.Xlibrispublishing.co.uk
Orders@Xlibrispublishing.co.uk
721533

MEDICAL HEALTH CENTRE

Disability support for the unwell and severely ill
Hospitality suite
Health clinic

Employees

Employees must be given several differing duties and tasks for their vocation including attending to the needs of patients and remaining alert to their requirements. They must handle duties professionally reserving the intent of their title. They must occupy them self with time to concentrate and get focused to deal with their occupation. A two page contract will be handed too employees for them too enrol and register with the company. All employees will be expected to complete a twenty page assignment of their profession and occupation in the use of a booklet manual for their acceptance anything before that will be provisional acceptance. A twenty page reference for perspective patients will add to the atmosphere of intelligence and security.

Doctors will be employed to keep records on patient check, as like any medical clinic they will prescribe medications and refer doctors to other patient clinics for assessment and various other therapies. Doctors will be expected to attend to sick elderly and disabled patients whilst researching their ailments, the paperwork they use for this will be publicised in health and safety manuals as well as posters on their wall.

Hospital hospitality wont is scarce in the hospital suite provided a warm kindness and generosity will be sent around the health clinic and assorted into day-by-day routine as stated on the medical file briefed in diagnostic assignments. Company policy contracts will be signed to the general staff to maintain this trend of activity. Staff in the clinic will be expected to take care of patients day and night.

Health centre the focus of health will be the main priority at the medical health centre; employees will be expected to enter employment with an established doctrine of professional studies showcasing their ability to occupy their advocated position as a doctor. A fifteen by eight point diagnostic assessment will take place weekly in the health centre; inductions will be critical for trainee therapist in their first year and mandatory.

Surgery clients will be treated by a duty therapist in a beauty chair or massage beds, these will have to be booked and all patients must have been checked by a nurse and seen by a doctor before consolidating therapy when in therapy they will be asked for a small fee and a term of payment whilst in surgery. Disabled patients are to receive devout treatment for their lively hood and benefit. In the surgery severely ill patients will receive the most beneficial service available form our doctors.

Consulting room patients will have to be consulted and diagnosed to see wither they are fit able or well enough to leave on going treatment, these files and records of treatment will be applied to the candidates records and reviewed whilst consulting.

Private clinic private assessment can be arranged for people who are severely ill with a private condition a team will then refer to an outpatients unit where you can find specified treatment. This is an exclusive community clinic any various signings will be referred to the national health service for support.

Treatment centre the medical health centre is a treatment building for people who are in need of some form of medication and who are irritably unwell. Support for the disabled and severely will be an issue looked at and relaxed upon the most frequently. Hospitality

MEDICAL HEALTH CLINIC A SOCIAL CARE GUIDE

arrangements for the ill and elderly will be a priority dealt with on a day-to-day basis.

Nurse keep a contingent affair with their clients and patients and make sure that they are treated until they are well enough for release. Also help claim any benefits or government grants.

Care for the necessity of a patient's health and don't become to involve with them research there past and find out the specifications of their illness and its origin. Nurses will have to research into the problems of their clients health and ensure they are well staff will be reminded to not become involved with their clients patents health.

Look after sick and elderly patients whilst in the surgery and ensure that they are hydrated recuperative and safe in their environment. Nurses are expected to be kind towards staff and patients responsible towards clients helpful to patients in their care and awaiting treatment and nurses must always remember to advocate for the disabled following this procedure with a warming smile.

Take care of clients and patients in their environment, on premises nurses will have the duty of taking care of clients and patients notes records registration and physical well being.

Tend to their ill health and physical mental needs and disabilities, monitor their health their symptom and their attributed health problems ensure they are in clarity have a full treatment assessment and that they wont get sick when you leave them.

Foster if patients have a problem or difficulty into their day-to-day basis nurses are expected to refer them to any demands they may have, such as housing rest bite or even re-creative activity. Take responsibility of a patient if they go into a seizure or incur fits and spasms. Advance a patient's daily life and ensure that they are meeting trademarks to get better by keeping them a good and prosperous social outlook.

Nurture nurse must assist their patients with a keen duty to order their self esteem and physical nourishment this means keep them up hydrated and tend to them continually for the duration of their ill health. This can relate to their dietary aspect or even their physical discomfort nurses must do, as their patients require. The health of patients is the first priority when a doctor or nurse is occupying the clinic, hygiene is paramount to the aid of patients getting well so this will be practiced with good continuity, cleanliness is a must, ailments and symptoms most be checked and assessed through out the stay of an unhealthy patient.

Paediatricians

Look after the care and treatment of kids

Monk a monk will be hired to take meditation classes and hose a department for company policy and staff management.

Priest a priest will be hired to assist with patients in the case of a burdened issue. The elderly will get special attention in particular by the priest who will sought them poetry and biblical mantras to keep them safe and calm just in case they become depressed or anxious at any stage.

Nun a nun will also be on the staff duty records or can be recorded as the main nurse who will be the sovereign manager of nurses insuring patients get the best treatment possible and that the company polices codes of conduct terms and conditions are making government requirement and that everything is in order.

Peaceful mind

At the medical health centre-calming music will be played on instrumental and air conditioners will be used in the main reception to keep customers happy.

Counsellor counselling will be top priority and the manager of the clinic will enrol with the local council with the intent of setting about fundamental intention. Then local council will be alerted to the workings of the medical health centre.

Therapist a therapist will work at the surgery to ensure that everything is going well for a patient. Their main duty will be to ensure that the progress of a patient's health is well treated and doesn't become unbalanced. Their will be a range of different therapist treating the disabled and unwell.

Psychotherapist a psychotherapist will be appointed to take care of patients who are mentally ill and in need of assistance in their day to day routine. If they are unsure of a patient or they appear to become continually unstable they will be expected to set them up with a referral scheme. Any illness will be given a therapeutic chair and diagnosed thoroughly as appropriate.

Psychoanalyst if problems are persistent and reoccurring a psychoanalysis will be asked to revise the health of a patient for further treatment with they are disabled elderly sick or at a young age. This will be done by a consultant for all sick injured and disabled patients.

Analysts will be down by the receptionist at the counter she will then refer the client to a consultant, who will do an analysis to diagnose them further. If a patient is found to have harmful symptoms then they will be seen by a doctor therapist immediately.

Shrink a shrink will release patients after their treatment has been performed if they are seen as well enough.

Consultant a consultant will run a diagnostic on the patient by using the correct body graphs and diagram charts. He will then instruct the patient on what they got to do to get better if the patient is seen as well enough to continue with treatment they will be referred onto another doctor who will prescribe them with medication.

Expert research constant evaluation and continuous observation will go into practice when taking care of clients, books articles journals and clearly decisive reports will be used to print further books and articles with loose distinction.

Specialist will be hired and recruited to treat various disease and problematic infections. Research on symptoms and ailments will be expected in the surgery and at the clinic round the clock whilst each patient is working, these procedures will be done in the form of assignments and diagnostics.

Professional certified staff would be hired and trained, those who do well at their vocations will have a better offering to advance in the hospitality carer. All doctors will be asked on assignment for their specified designations as a therapist, these doctors and nurses will be graded on their evaluation and a decision of independence will be given at the end of each working year.

Authority will be given to the manager of department in the form of council duty; this will be in the form of company policy permission sheets and staff contracts.

Advisor a health advisor will be on hand to advise patients of anything if they're having any problems. (Terms conditions requirements codes of practice)

Mentor a mentor will help clients with any problems and keep them activated reminding them to have a balance of innovation and health.

Guide a guide will be about to help any patients with a distressing issue, if they are in need of refereed counselling a guide can help them with this.

Dieticians a dietician chef will be on duty to cook and prepare meals twenty four hours a day for ill and disabled patients who are in need of a nutritional meal placement four their dietary health supplement. These cooks will reserve time to discuss their clients nutritional vitals and what meal they need to support them further.

MEDICAL HEALTH CLINIC A SOCIAL CARE GUIDE

Health expert a health expert will be put in charge of doctors and nurses reports files and findings through this they will train staff and employees on what support clients need for various ailments. These health experts will be on hand for publication of illustrated photographed diagnostics and various other methods of staff training and development.

Cleaners will be hired to run daily duties to see that the ecology of the unit remains healthy and friendly. They ill be assigned shifts to work round the clock sanitizing and keeping the buildings interior clean safe tidy and perfectly presented. The duty of the cleaners will be on an agriculture contract for the ecology of cleaners.

Hygiene attendants these cleaners will ensure that the hygiene and cleanliness of the unit is completely well and orderly.

Sanitizers will be used in a range of clinical methods form eucalyptus plants to honey dew resin mixed in a spray canister. They will be dispensed to the cleaning staff and made the focus of cleaning up grimy areas for the sake of community hygiene and clarity.

Secretaries will be hired to arrange files at reception take and make phone calls keep appointments register staff and employees.

Bookkeepers will ensure that contract registration and enrolment is conducted to a professional standard. Contact government bodies and get involved with community links and partnerships. Study market research making appointments with clientele for mergers. (Work closely with administration to get finance arranged and certified)

Administration

Registration – in order to have the likelihood of treatment at the medical health centre you will need to make arrangements to register your details and the duty receptionist will refer to one of our doctors.

Fees – in order to maintain a productive balance a manageable monthly fee will be expected by patients this will then go to their overall treatment at the medical health centre.

Partnerships – will be based on health and hospitality organisations regarding the references of patient's illnesses and the type of health they need to seek out.

Contracts - contracts will be handled by the receptionist for patients staff contracts will be handled on the professionals file who will then adhere to the terms and conditions of contract.

Advantages

Better care then hospitals

At the medical health centre patient treatments will be more friendly and negotiable their will be no uncleanness smells or bad hygiene all doctors and nurses will be on call to treat patients twenty four hours a day.

Three square meals will be provided a day to keep the vitality of patients up registered care will be taken to stop further ailments being met with patients.

Showers and baths will be available once a patient is seen as fit they will be required to leave and in the worst case scenario escorted to a different hospital for further treatment.

Safer treatment

Treatment will be looked into to cure and test for a number of different ailments and treatments.

A range of different methods will be available without the use of a needle or Machinery a polite decency will be shown to all patients and safety procedures will be taken to prevent any other problem from showing up.

Happier staff and patients

Staff will ensure that a comfortable distance is kept between them and their patients company socialising and restraint will go hand in hand giving the staff a stable hand in dealing with their patients.

Staff will ensure that patients receive the correct advice and information on problematic health and deal with an extensive range of curing ill symptoms

More stable community

The health benefits and safety measures produced by the medical health centre will be improvisation

The administration of the medical health centre will be treated as a hospital type contract, position will be past and a funding committee will make sure registrations have the correct referendum for funding.

Through different schemes and health meetings the community will gather a stable health.

Booklets and hard-copies will be sold on sight in the doctors to give to customers and patients in the community explaining health and safety methods.

Stable income

More employment activity will open up better jobs for the community will give way to a stabile society.

Worthwhile treatment The options available will be vast and far more advanced and safer then modern hospitals.

Overall well being of patient health and safety

When patients come into the care of the medical health centre they will have their details registered and a small fee applied.

All accidents and injuries will be taken to note on their medical file without lengthy disruptions or irritations.

All medical and treatment will be given and advanced and civil look. A team of trustworthy will handle overnight treatment and eligible nurses who will ensure that everyone is in good condition.

Better hygiene

Hygiene and cleanliness will be provided continually without the use of peroxide and other unfriendly chemical waste.

More advanced holistic medication care

Advanced holistic medical care will be on the agenda for more suitable and viable symptom care atoning symptoms and managing the ailments of sick patients relieving them from poor health.

Better researched symptoms and a more advanced arrangement of hospitality

At the medical centre arrangements will be made for medical staff examination theory and diagnostic induction tests.

We will be ensuring that our staff are properly trained and guided on the standards of solving and administrating to the care of subjects and patients.

Hospitality guidance will be issued to staff on training periods were they will be assigned the task of initiating different theoretically related health checks.

Diagnostics will be set in accordance to standards and provision of work to check on the capability of therapy staff.

With guidelines paperwork and symptom safety methods staff will work to a professional standard to ensure the health and safety of patients.

More stable employment in the economy

The weight of the medical centre will house to gain roughly 250 employees at a time ranging in a number of different practices.

The training methods and induction traditions will bring about out going and civilised activities around the community making the community a more stable place to live.

MEDICAL HEALTH CLINIC A SOCIAL CARE GUIDE

Increased chance of recreation

The poster corner will be attended to regularly and given a good outlook of reference for the improvisation of recreation.

Exercise will be the forecast for patients who have taken ill due to poor circulation and lack of activity. This poster corner will be revised and put up with many different office statements.

Hire standards of good living

People will be able to return to their daily lives well and unharmed the symptom relief and medication provided would support and keep people on top of their health.

A maintenance check ups and good service will be high on the agenda professional staff will look after and ensure the health to the community is maintained unless a case is refereed then the medical health centre pulls out and leaves the case up to another team.

More options in injuries and accidents

The medical health team are not like usual hospital staff. They have moral hygiene and their surgeries have advanced practitioners and they don't use the unhygienic method of needles to oversee accidents and injuries.

Options are available for people when they come in with an injury to see a nurse who will attend to their wound with water and lemon cress.

Advanced patient health checks

Health checks will be handled by therapists doctors and nurses these will be reviewed at monthly intervals looking for any problems and diagnosis if any thing seems wrong or the patient is healthy they are seen as fit to leave.

Occupations — staff are expected to occupy themselves in the surgery on their working hours by

Work with disabled

At the medical health centre the staff will be expected to work with the disabled intensely to ensure that their needs are met. Working with the disabled is top priority at the medical health centre.

Attend to the unwell

Doctors and nurses are expected to work with the unwell and not what their doing if they do not qualify for working with the unwell then they will not be expected to attend the medical centre for employment.

Make medication

Therapy staffs are expected to make suitable and viable medication for the patients and always have a bright eye and a bushy tail.

Give health and safety hygiene advice

When working for the medical health centre staff will be expected to review health and safety symptoms for booklets and commission panels so they will be well inducted and expected to know a range of different therapeutic advice so they can give appropriate health and safety advice to their patients.

Cure symptoms

Doctors will be expected to cure symptoms with haste and to an advanced rationality healing various wounds and treating differing health problems.

Arrange appointments

A receptionist will be on hand to arrange different appointments and ensure that patients are receiving the correct doctor as well as consultants who will provide a knowledgeable diagnosis who will then refer you to an appropriate therapist who will then cure the patient's symptom.

Compile booklets

Doctors and nurses will train under intense supervision of a specialist doctor who will instruct them on how to be professional in medical care they will all be then expected to compile booklets form research examples.

Look after patients

All medical; staff will have a retrospective duty too look after patients and ensure their care is provided with patients and restraint they will also be expected not get to occupied attached or personnel with patients and staff unless training socialising or gaining companionship.

Ensure the are nourished and hydrated

When patients make a choice to stay overnight or for a time period they will be expected to make sure that patients get registered and are looked after by feeding them three square meals a day.

Cure and revise illness's

Consultants will work in close links to cure and revise illness's ensuring that everything is taken care off and that they are not showing any symptoms.

Make sure that all is safe and well with clientele

Consultants will have the duty o ensuring that everything is kept to a fair understanding with patients showing a polite demeanour adhering to the responsibilities expected at a medical centre.

Maintain cleanliness' and clarity of rooms better hygiene

Dieticians are too looking after the balanced diet and detoxify of patients advising them on what food to eat.

Consultants are to ensure that patients are seen to after the have spoke to a receptionist, the consultant will then refer them to a specified nurse/doctor who will see that the their patient needs are meet.

A massage therapist will be called in to ensure that the comfort ability and physique of a patient is in good order.

Nurses will be ask to perform regular health checks on customers and register patients monthly to ensure that there blood pressure and overall health is in good condition.

A well trained and high briefed holistic therapist will make sure that medication is produced and dispensed for specific patients using ph balance and body function scales.

Hydrotherapy will be dispensed to people who are severely ill but only if they are severely ill as hydrotherapy is a highly reserved treatment. A hydro therapist is a practitioner who ensures that everyone is well and vital stabilising critical and fundamental health.

Meditation sessions will be available for those who are suffering mental illness these will be formed in special classes and will be arranged by the topic of a mental health counsellor.

Disabled physiotherapy top priority for the medical health centre disabled physiotherapy is a doctor's occupation a qualified doctor will review the health of a severely disabled patient and gradually nurse them back to health. This treatment will be down over an advanced and lengthy period.

The medical centre will have a nurse who looks for symptoms on a ph graph avoiding needles and other unpleasant bad practices. These ph graphs will be used on a regular basis for health checks and relevant illness diagnostics.

Symptoms will be analysed and reviewed by a practitioner who will ensure that the correct treatment is provided. A range of studies will be expected to be studied using ph graphs and body diagrams to alleviate poor symptoms accurately.

A holistic therapist who will mix and prescribe a mixture of different herbs and antibiotics will handle medication cared.

Hygiene will be on the company polices and handled by a list of different doctors and nurses the surgery areas and patient rooms will be clean all of the time. Cleaning and sanitising their area of work regularly on a daily basis.

The over all well being of staff and patients will be looked at and reviewed secretaries and administration will ensure that everybody is registered and given a monthly review to ensure good practice. Paper research reports documents meetings articles relating to the importance of health and safety.

Paediatrician

Health

Support for the bodies vitality

At the medical centre we will offer support for the well being of the bodies vitality, taken car of unhealthy symptoms and treating vital growth and muscular improvements.

More cause for recreation and positive activity

Leaflets and various posters will be posted in reception to remind clients of treatments for ailments and various other symptoms, given advice and incentive to regular patients as well as any community schemes.

Better nutrition for the weak and disabled and the ill treated

Health diet and food advice will be available for overnight patients as well as health food specialists. Nurture patients that come into their care supporting their nutritional needs and valuing their word.

Cured treatment will lead to a more integral innovative community

The doctors and nurses will be specialising in rehabilitating poor health and meeting requirements. After a patient is seen as fit they will be given a clean bill of health and sent away from the premises until they feel ill again.

Healthier hygiene from hydrotherapy

Hygiene will be taken care of through nursing and hospitality hydrotherapy will be used for people suffering from severe exhaustion.

Healthier physique from physiotherapy

Physiotherapy will be used most commonly for the disabled unless an able body person such as a sportsman or women takes ill they can book an appointment. Physiotherapist will be dedicated to the health of a disabled person.

Healthier minds from meditation

A monk will be appointed to run a class.

Hygiene

trained cleaners that well ensure that rooms are cleaned and sanitised throughout the day.

Sickness common hospitals have poor hygiene, which leads to a desperation of health, these desperations cause sickness at the medical health centre.

Sickness is expected to be scarce and unlikely as the buildings hygiene is revised and asserted twenty-four hours a day by a team of sanitising doctors and nurses who specialise in the treatment go bad hygiene.

Bad hygiene from sickness is caused when a person lacks clarity or observation skills in practising cleaning them.

If someone doesn't wash himself or herself after performing in the toilet or having an open wound accident then their sickness will continue due to the fact of their bad hygiene.

Clinical methods have to be performed without the use of metals, which convey the long-term characteristics of excrement to avoid sickness through bad hygiene.

Hygiene must be dealt with by using negotiable practices such as wet rags and clean appliances there is no way you cant sought hygiene through metal it makes the hygiene worse.

MEDICAL HEALTH CLINIC A SOCIAL CARE GUIDE

Hygiene can also make the problems of ill health better you without worrying about sickness and the spread germs and keeping on top of your hygiene you can stay out of the way pf ill health.

Health is attributing to hygiene especially in the case of eating well and washing your hands before a meal it is also important to remember that if you do not sanitise your meal before you eat the hygiene from your meal can cause you to be come ill.

These symptoms could lead to an unhealthy decay and the spread of bacteria germs all of this will be reviewed and advised by a health doctor.

Staying on top of your hygiene or if you are crippled finding a good place to make your hygiene better is imperative.

This could be in the form of washing regularly and eating the correct balance, fruit and a well-designated radox bath could be the best thing for you to stay on the top of your hygiene.

The physical condition and vigour of your hygiene is the main attribute of your health's sanitation regular exercise and a good wash can help to create the perfect balance of your hygiene overall health.

Ability is sometimes an issue for people when taking care of their health these people usually need support.

Disabled people taken care of their hygiene may not be able to access their necessities to do this so it is important that they have twenty-four hour assistance.

Having the ability to take care and respond to your hygiene is an important factor so if your lazy or just idle then you don't need hospital treatment.

People with sever illness or more important to attend to in this instance so it is important to enrol and register any disabilities so that a specialist nurse or doctor can be assigned to you for twenty-four a day assistance.

Apart from a sever disability there is no reason why you cant take care of your hygiene people with bad hygiene show the worst case of symptom.

These people will have to make arrangements for other care facilities as company policy states that by no order can a monotonous standard make a claim or register with the medical health centre.

Clarity is important to maintain a clearness of hygiene will keep you prompted from unwell hazard.

When people are looking clarity and they hygiene that need to find a suitable way to wash. If clarity is kept and maintained then the body's ambiguity can be distinctive.

Cleanliness washing frequently and without lackey incentive or the use of perversion. Cleaning yourself in general in cleaning yourself just to meet occasion, doing this will make people enjoy your company and be happy 6tovhave you around.

Disability support

A range of therapies will be available for people with sever disabilities, they will be prioritised and attended to continually through out the day.

The therapies available to them will be top of the range and systemically available, a reserve of therapeutic counselling and maintained balance of night-time assistance by a twenty-four hour appointed therapeutic nurse.

The therapies available to the disabled will be therapeutic and authorized intensely for the maintenance of the disabled patients healthy balance.

MEDICAL HEALTH CLINIC A SOCIAL CARE GUIDE

Continued and focused nursing for a disabled person round the clock duty will be offered the duties nurse will be enlisted to take on the agenda of the disabled clients care needs a risk assessment will be taken and advised offered.

The hygiene and protection of the disabled client will be aided in every way possible, their diet will be adjusted and peace of mind kept by a cognizant therapeutic nurse.

Hydration therapy and the best of service will be approached with our disabled clients.

Constant research to find a cure for the impaired anatomy a doctor in the surgery will be referred too the disabled client to investigate their case and living standards.

This doctor will then research the anatomy of their illness in order to find a cure for the disability in the form of ailment symptom or disability rehabilitation treatment.

Consistent counselling from the highest of authority at the medical health centre will be the direct register priority given to by the disabled.

BUSINESS PLAN

Rooms

Over twenty different patients check rooms throughout the building housing local patients.

Hospitality room for visitors staff and patients, were a buffet will be served and people get the correct supplement.

Employment more people will be employed for their profession, their vocations will be checked on certification standard and probation assignment contract (work experience)

Economics there will be more stable opportunities for health and people in the community.

Nutrition will be on the agenda for the medical health centre medical check on people who enrol as patients.

Health will be incorporated into the environment were people occupy surgery rooms pie chart and food graphs displaying different health check methods.

Safety will be advised and study frequently by the on duty doctors who will be lending their initiative and certification to the establishment of medical health diagnosis.

Innovation will be displayed in the rooms showing different patients who enter the room how well their vocation is doing at what the can do to occupy themselves.

Food will be available also in the form of fruit and meal tickets given to the sick patients who will be expected to pay monthly registration fees for their premium.

Diet will be ordered by the doctor on these occasions and arranged by assessment and prescription by the counter.

Recreation will be analysed by a paediatrician and a health expert who will be authorised via consultant at the clinic.

Vitality will be assessed in the rooms by a various assortment of diagnosis equipment
That will check to measure your health's instability.

Occupied by hard-working professionals

Hard working professionals and consultants will work in these rooms twenty for hours a day with the help of a hygiene nurse and a medical doctor ensuring that everything is well and safe.

Cleaned and sanitised after every patient use

Hygiene nurses will clean and sanitise the buildings safety working for the beneficial progress of clarity and cleanliness.

Furnishings

Beds a number of beds will be bought for overnight staff and patients who have booked a room, usually this will be for the disabled and only ill people are allowed to stay in them.

Mattress will be cleaned and maintained by keen staff members employed to sanitise and clean the linen.

Sheets will be the main focus of a cleaner's duty, they will be efficient cleaned and tidied after each use and they must remain cleanly for the use of patients.

Specialist pillows specially shaped and buffed pillows will be arranged and made for the use patients and clients who suffer disabilities they will be arranged and ordered to meet their needs for an overnight stay.

Vases will be in the surgery with plants put into them they will be their for the continuity of the rooms patients who will find that they make the air cleaner to breath.

Bathtubs will be in the surgery rooms for people who are ill for therapy these will be used for disabled clients and those who are appointed by a consultant for therapy treatment.

Posture chairs these will be put in the reception patient waiting area for the use of visitor's clients and patients these posture chairs will be for the promotional use of physical health.

Massage tables will be purchased for the use of massage therapist and the conditioning of the physical health of patents they will be put into a therapy doctor's room and used for the treatment of ill patients.

Flooring will be decided upon and used by the hire arrangements of renovators who will renovate the floor with pine flooring.

Beauty cabin a beauty cabin will be used to store and treat clients with ill health symptom medication and ailment advice will be available in these stores.

Chiropody cabin health and safety tools will be stored in here as well as a doctor's kit and special routine.

Trolleys will be on display taken medication and food around to patients throughout the clinic.

Paperwork will be handled and filed by staff and employees in their surgery room these will be handled contingent and lightly in the form of notes and distinctive records to avoid clarity.

Tables will be supplied for the use of resting items in the reception area for visitors and patients.

Chairs will be in the lobby area also for the use of sitting their will be roughly twelve chairs available in the form of sofas for a comfortable seating arrangements.

Kitchens utensils these will be used in the kitchen area and by a health chef who will cook and prepare meals according to diet for patients.

Refurbishment this will be down on entrance of business the building will get a healthier interior and a more designated out look to the buildings current state.

Office the reception will be treated as an office, were people are expected to work and file notes. The company manager will work on site and ensure that staff and employees are meeting targets and complying with company policies.

Desk a desk will be stored in nurse and doctor rooms were various cabinets and health stencils will be occupant a phone and various other commodities will come with this.

Storage cabinet a storage cabinet will be purchased and put in a convenient place for the use of doctors and nurses.

Tools/equipment

Respiratory diagrams
B-m-I monitor a body monitor will be used on patients in the doctor's room to check their blood pressure.

This will be stored on the side of the desk and be for doctor and medical use only, the body mass will then go on their files for medical evidence and health conditions.

If they pass a certain level from their diagnosis they won't be able to qualify for their treatment.

Ph balance chart a red too white ph balance chart will be stored in the doctor's surgery and used by all the staff on site when inclined to run testing on patients.

This will be in the form of a two hundred centre metre strip colour balance paper and be used to review the colour balance in the acid alkaline of a patient predetermine the illness of patients.

Body graphs body graphs will be drawn in the form of body points and charted on the surgery rooms, these body graphs will be distinct body physique and indicate which structures of the body are most liable to pain. Patients will then consult were to mark of the burdened area for the doctor to give them distinct advice about their treatment.

First aid bag a first aid bag will be the duty of the nurse this will be stored in their cabinet the use will be instructed by a nun who will decide how to use the first aid on patients these will consist on a stethoscope torch Vento ling inhaler bandages wet wipes and various other medical equipment.

Hygiene gloves hygiene gloves will be available in the surgery room and accompanied by sanitised water bottles, these will be for the use of patients who have an open wound or and injury of some sought. (Absence treatment.)

Bedding cabinet a bedding cabinet will be stored in sleepover rooms and be for the specific use of cleaners on sanitising duty to keep fresh clean and well buffed continually all the time.

MEDICAL HEALTH CLINIC A SOCIAL CARE GUIDE

Plastic beverage retainers these will be supplied and stored by the chef who will ensure that every meal is served freshly and to the satisfaction of hygiene and clarity.

Plastic beverage retainers will be used and washed regularly to avoid the threat of spreading infections.

Nursing records nursing records will be kept in a file for the use of a nurse, these nurses will do extensive research and at the end of each month write a theory document of their occupation until they have reached a high level in their occupation.

Blood pressure monitors these will be stored in the surgery and used on patients to check for any blood abnormalities and wither they patient has any blood conditions.

Doctor's diagnostic kit a diagnosis kit will be similar to the nurse's bag except it has doctors paraphernalia instead usually attribute to their qualification.

Patient's blankets Nurse's kit these will be supplied to the nurses whilst on twenty-four hour care duty looking after patients on call.

Medicines

Holistic medicine will be revised and grown in a garden; these will then be extracted in a laboratory.

Were they will be dispensed to clients in the form of medication this could be as pills or as tea bags usually to relieve symptoms.

Drugs will be prescribed to severely ill patients who will then have to take them over a varied amount of time to get better.

Once their drug intake medication term is expired a consultant who will assess them for further treatment will review them.

Remedies will be prescribed to patients who are severely in need of an antidote for their sickness this remedy will then be dispensed top them via the specified doctor who will recommend a dose and set time to take them.

Tablets will be prescribed to patients who are suffering from any mental illnesses these will be for patients who are in serious need of relaxation.

Tablets and amphetamines or for relaxation purposes and should only be taken if patients are in need of a serious laxative.

Pills will be processed with solution water and scented minerals for the use of poor conditions.

The people who take these pills will get their prescription from this surgery in particular.

Herb will be grown the medical facility and analysed by a holistic doctor for use of medicinal purposes, the practitioner will research the cause of symptom and effect of the herb.

Aromatic plant these will be for the use of aromatherapy, these plants will be located in the nursing rooms and allocated to the therapists for treatment purposes.

Florists will be linked to the medical centre were they will grow special herbs and balms for the use of medicinal purposes.

Diet will be served to sick patients for their nutrient value along with their vitality; a diet doctor will be hired to revise the health of a patient's illness and dietary imbalance.

Food will only be served to patients in order to aid their health dietary requirements will be reviewed and the specified requirements will be their to balance the clients health.

Nutrition the dietician will decide on the level of nutrition needed to get their patients back to a good level of health.

Meals will be prepared round the clock and be specific of what the patient needs; if the patient is being taken care of in a room then they will be giving three square meals a day.

Massage will be available to treat patients who are in need of chiropody or wither they are suffering from any physical condition.

A doctor who will other a therapeutic treatment to a patient and analyse to see if they need a nurse to treat them for their melancholy symptom will consult depression.

A massage therapist who will gibe regular sessions until the muscle ach has gone comfortably and with one hundred per cent symmetry will treat muscle ach.

Poor physique if a client is suffering from poor physique their illness will be diagnosed by a doctor who will assess them for therapeutic treatment.

Sports therapy when sports men/women register with medical health clinic they will be given monthly inductions if they are active as sportsman for a regular massages health check.

Aroma will be used to maintain the clarity and hygiene of patients if they receive treatment and show no improvements they will be turned away form the surgery and deemed as indecent.

Sensible hygiene methods will be instructed by the counsellor if they are not meet and the counsellors sees the patient as nauseating, then the counsellor has the right refuse them permission to re-enter the establishment.

Purchased products will be extracted form a garden stored in a laboratory and purchased in regular shops.

A consultant who will take it into their hands will apply for soap conditioning to treat patients they will then prescribe it to them and instruct them on how to use it.

Smell detoxification if a client is point five unhygienic then they will be required to undergo a smell detoxification before they are considered for further treatment.

Eye examination. If their eye condition is tragic then they will be An eye doctor who will run an eye diagnosis on the health of a client patient's retina will conduct treatment if the retina is poor this will be in the form of prescribed glasses or eye treatment.

Retinas scans will be available for client patients who are in need of further treatment a consultant will take their review into account and ensure that they are fair and well.

Blood sugar will be looked for in surgical procedures a doctor will diagnose a patient by the standards of their blood pressures activity.

Ph balance the red to white balance of patient's ailments will be stored and revised for acid to alkali symptom in the patients system.

Vital strength this will be reviewed and analysed by the nature of the health problem and assessed.

The ability of the patient's vitals should reflect the area of sickness causing symptom in patients.
Diet efficiency will be reviewed and revised by the assessment of the dietician, when the dietician has finished the assessment the dietician will then food graph the nourishment needed for the patients health restoration.

Physical health of a patients well being well be looked at and revised if they are ill through ailment then a physical body graph will assess symptom.

If their sickness is causing problems in the mental compartment then sleep methods will be consulted.

Temperature will be taken and measured without the use of a thermometer the illness will be handled by feeling the problems relating to the ill health of a patients body.

Cold fever warm fever regular frostbite irregular frostbite allergy symptom strength management.

Fever is the fever intoxicating the patient what is the cause of intoxication, is the fever felt by the patient leading to a permanent syndrome, what effects are concurrent in the fever of the patient what is the best way to find their cure.

Hydration can be the effect of a poor symptom that leads to a temperamental fever simple methods of taking care of the clients hydration and liquidation can do a lot to help with preventing the client to become ill any further.

Physical ability can also be stagnant if a temperature is extremely serious, if the physical ability of a patient is extremely unbalanced by their temperature then a few recovery methods may be vital for the stability of a patience health.

Ailment will be arranged if a patients temperature or condition is worsening they will be given the efficient supplement to keep them aware and until their conditions are bettered.

Hydration is important for the vitality of the bodies immune system and active ability
Vitality in this case will come in the form of liquid water for nourishment.

This hydrating nourishment will be used for patients who are severely ill with a problematic condition.

As long as they didn't do it to themselves then they will be given suitable treatment until they are well again.

Life vitals will have to be measured and recorded for the patient to adjust and get the correct treatment this could be in the form of soup or just a place to rest whilst the nurse helps you with any symptoms that you may be undergoing.

Mental stamina can also be a problematic effect cased by patients who have suffered from dehydration.

When the stamina is lost it can usually come from a traumatic experience that disrupts the mental ability of the body's energy stagnant energy.

With this problem it would be important for the patients to seek advice on their medical treatment.

Movement will be difficult so a resolution will have to be made for the support of the patients needs.

Ability can be a problematic experience energy spasms and a lack of endurance that may need constructive activity.

Sanity can be poorly effected by a patient suffering from hydration as the body functions shut down after hydration is needed the mental sanity of a patient can be put at risk if they lack this hydration.

A consultant and the patient's assigned doctor who will give the patient medical advice and a medication prescription for a specified amount of time will handle symptom analysis the symptom analysis of patent medicinal benefits.

Daily pattern will be reviewed and revised by a consultant for the analysis of a patient's health problems and best type of medication.

Standards of routine if a client has difficulty with their routine then they will be assigned a special nurse who will give them twenty four support.

Disability treatments. Will be on hand and the key theme of the medical health centres objective.

MEDICAL HEALTH CLINIC A SOCIAL CARE GUIDE

Disabled clientele will have the option of treatment freely and with fair and orderly advice.

Once deemed as the disabled and properly registered the disabled person will have fair and permanent treatment all with the intention of getting well.

Round the clock assistance will be high on the agenda for the people with lack of ability they will be given all the help needed, from a clean and sanitised living condition to hydrotherapy and aroma therapy.

Physiotherapy will be in order for the care and recuperation of the disabled client who will be given special physiotherapy treatment to cure their condition.

Nurse doctor care the terms and conditions of nurse and doctor staff will be to take care of the ill patients needs and ensure that they are comfortable in their care as well as making sure they are getting better.

Oxidation
Mandatory teenage check up
The detoxification of ill bones (teeth)
The hygiene of a patient's respiratory system

Consultant therapies

Expert doctors will be on hand to lend advice to patients on wither or not they are healthy enough to undergo patient therapies.

If the patient is seen as too healthy the consultant therapist will turn them, away and advice them too look after the health in their own. In any case the consultant therapist is in the highest chain of command from all of the other doctor and nurse therapists.

The monk who has a high stake in the medical organisation will teach breathing therapy he will run classes on the breathing and exercise of patients.

Dietician medication detoxifies nutrition supplement food groups all of these will be on the list of agenda for the running of the medical health centres facilities.

Doctors nurses and consultants will be hired to manage and maintain the standards of this in their company policies if they fell to meet the standards and policies expected of them their employment will be terminated and contracts stopped.

Hydration therapies medical hydration this is a very special therapy and is only to be used by people who are suffering from serious deliriousness or in a difficult situation with their vital health.

Aromatherapies health and hygiene aroma this is only for patients who are enrolled and undergoing special treatments, if a registered patient asks for this treatment they will have to apply and they will be refereed to a further employment were they will be expected to pay a small fee.

Massage therapy acupuncture coalescence alleviation these will be given to patients who are in particular need of treatment. These treatments will be performed after a patient has been reviewed.

Specialist
Physiotherapy
For the disabled intensive therapies
For the severely ill
On special demand

As the medical centre is specifically for the disabled they will get special treatment throughout their period of sickness and taken cared of for whatever sickness they are paying for.

Mergers will be made in the local community to suit the needs of conservative people. These mergers will go to the stable development of client patient care and the best part of referrals.

National Health Service merger: people will be instructed to refer to us through different members of the National Health Service who

MEDICAL HEALTH CLINIC A SOCIAL CARE GUIDE

will direct them into or care if they are seriously ill or physically wounded.

General practitioner practice merge: general practitioner service will refer their patients to our care if necessary in any case the general practitioner will have us on file.

Local council merge: funds will be applied for as a business foundation from the local council who will receive our intelligence on different types of illness's and ways of treating ailments.

Housing service merge: nurses will be on call and on duty round the clock twenty four hours to deal with any seriously ill patients in need of a house call or twenty four seven assistance.

Advocates avocations will be the registration and association apparent in society for community members to register and councils to join as members.

Community members advocated: members of the community will be advocated to work in the medical health centre and through engage in special activities such as fun days and yearly festivals.

Housing services advocated: patients who arrive ill or homeless will be given shelter until a form of accommodation can be provided for them, when this accommodation is found the medical health centre will contribute to three months worth of rent or help provide the mortgage.

Nurse staff nurse's duty advocated: nurses will be expected to take a mature outlook with their patients and help them out of rude illness so a lot of patients and humility will be required of such nurses.

Most nurses will be expected two work twenty four seven and remain dutiful except for breaks and shift changes.

On call doctors advocated: and on call doctor will be available for patients all day around the clock. The will attend to patients and be allocated in the health centre.

Holistic therapies advocated: special herbs spices and antibiotics will be made for the medication of patient's health and safety will be revised constantly building manuals and merchandising medical books for the benefit of other hospitals around the nation.

Twenty-four hour patient advice clinics advocated: round the clock hospitality will be available but only for patients who are sincerely severely ill with either injury or ailment.

Those who are sincerely sick and in need of hospitality advocated: no one will be allowed into the hospital unless they are generally ill and suffering from some form of illness.

If people walk in to the hospital claiming ill without any verified check up ailments they will be warranted off the premises.

Mental health doctors advocated: mental health doctors will also be available to consult with members of the public looking for the worries of their illness.

Hm revenue advocated: as a sole trader I will consult with the bank on getting a property.

then consult with hm revenues on getting charity and business registered shortly after I will get certified.

then shortly after that accredited once I am accredited I will higher employees with the intention of contracting them too statuary pay.

Certified accredited contracts will be referred to by the bank, building society job-centre or even the educational authority's grants and award scheme.

MEDICAL HEALTH CLINIC A SOCIAL CARE GUIDE

Contracts/Benefits
Statuary pay

Registered membership

Monthly fee

Accredited contract

Specially paid for treatment

Regular check-ups

Affective advice

Professional health options

Customers

Those who are severely sick and in need of medical attention

Registered patients who have an irregular illness

Injury patients who want normal procedures
Project statement
References will be assorted and bought forward too look for foundation links and various clientele in the local community and about the region.
The bank
HM revenues
Home office
National health service
Education services
Local general practitioners
Dentist
Farmers association
Town council

Details of address phone numbers fax machines will be arranged to make contact with these references particularly in the local community

Certification will be applied for via the government and given an accepted qualification stamp for the use of registered employment and company legislation rules.

Various paperwork such as contracts finance forms will be written up to report to type format then sent of certification and approval to the business standards agency.

Vocational assignments, such as the term of profession that employees have been assigned too will be typed up on staff training periods and sent off fro certification.

Qualified staff only will be employed here so a college course will be set up on the side to get them up to their qualification.

Accreditation will be looked for and vouched by administration via references and various money associations.

Accreditation will come from official money managers and authorised lenders. Endorsements will be expected from the National Health Service and various other money arranging organisations.

The bank

Employment contracts will be written up and given too staff for their terms of work and conditions of pay.

Applications will be handled on curriculum vitae covering letters must be bought forward as well as a copy of a ten thousand-word health therapy assignment for all applicants accepted.
    When the applicants receive their inductions they will have to make a choice of vocation on the employment contracts.

Enrolment

MEDICAL HEALTH CLINIC A SOCIAL CARE GUIDE

Company contracts will be illustrated and shown to clientele who will be given friendly advice and suitable options of how they will like to hold a steak in the company.

Company polices will be stated and written on the walls for staff and clients to read a like in very brief mandatory statements.

Patients

Staff

Clinic

Management

National Health Service

Education services

Registration

Employees

Financial arrangements

Community links

Company polices

Contracts

Markets

Local community

Local paper

Registration membership fees

Sick

Elderly

Disabled

Aims

Cure the sick

Treat the disabled

Comfort the elderly

Get rid of bad hygiene and spectroscope

Objectives

Maintain occupied and well duty staff

Benefit the community with employment and health options

Seek out appropriate retirement for the elderly
Cleanse and clarify the health of people

Stable finance

Obtaining finance

Registration

Membership

National Health Service

MEDICAL HEALTH CLINIC A SOCIAL CARE GUIDE

Agenda

Cash flowchart forecast
Pay
Earnings
Administration
Property
Equipment
Furnishings
Rooms
Employees
Staffs
Renovations
Refurbishments
Obtaining finance
Registration
Membership
National Health Service

Administration

Registration – in order to have the likelihood of treatment at the medical health centre you will need to make arrangements to register your details and the duty receptionist will refer to one of our doctors.

Fees – in order to maintain a productive balance a manageable monthly fee will be expected by patients this will then go to their overall treatment at the medical health centre.

Partnerships – will be based on health and hospitality organisations regarding the references of patient's illnesses and the type of health they need to seek out.

Contracts - contracts will be handled by the receptionist for patient's staff contracts will be handled on the professionals file who will then adhere to the terms and conditions of contract. A contract is a legal document between two parties a sole trader and a staff member, an employer and an employee this legal document binds them in division and work provision. Social security statuary pay income tax and vat must be attributed to the employee's contract when starting work to avoid any illegal legislation relating to administration of earning. A contract sets out in black and whites the rules and regulations that both parties agree to. Employer sets out rules and regulations on a contract and the employee is expected to comply or else they'll face immediate dismissal. Employer contract if a sole trader asks a staff or company member too work for a certain amount of hours this is a term and condition of contract. The term of the contract will be how long they work and the condition of contract is what they are expected to do a contract must be distinctive of two pages.

Registration

Accreditation

Employment

Earnings

Administration

Certification

Legislation

Statuary pay

Benefits Social security number

National insurance

Previous employer

Social security number

Rooms - 10 rooms in over ten leisure houses across the area will be erected. A min motel area tea girl motel will have all the amenities and luxuries of a regular hotel in a more compressed space with the added touch of elegance and spaciousness.

Jacuzzi – big bathtubs will be stored at the top of the restaurant in the gymnasium area were diners are welcome to book an appointment to get a massage from one of the hydration nurses. Pine floors will be renovated for a natural pan erotic look making the décor more therapeutic for the vocation of Jacuzzi room treatment. These appointments will be booked for diners who are willing to pay the extra cash for their meal.

Radox spa – in the radox spa specially scented water will be mixed for relaxation these will be done by an holistic therapist who will mix and experiment in a number of flowers and plant herbs these will be then stored in a doctors cabinet were they may be distributed to various pharmaceuticals.

Aromatherapy – appointments to see an aroma therapist will be made and kept this aroma therapist will bath you in scented oils and specially made candles.

Massage spa and acupuncture - Massage therapist will be key in rebalancing people and ensuring health spa facilitations are concordant.

Leisure arena - leisure arenas will be on hand for the use of exercise and workouts. these arenas will be a vital asset.

Caribbean menu – food will be served in the lower part of the diner this food will be from a range of different cultures, Caribbean food will be on the menu and a special chef will be on hand to take orders and write the menu. The five food groups will be put into the menus order marking the restaurant with a certified distinction. Foods such as starch potatoes rice, fruit tomatoes grapes, diaries cheese egg, vegetables sprouts broccoli, and protein meat carbohydrate meat fish chicken.

Oriental menu – an oriental menu will be served also these recipes will be from the orient and served for the enjoyment of customers.

Spanish menu – Spanish food will also be available from the restaurant this food is rear in this country and will go down a treat.

Kitchen equipment – an oven will be purchased, a cooker will be purchased, utensils will be purchased, a refrigerator will be purchased, cutlery will be purchased, pots and pans will be purchased, these will be priced up and put onto the cash flow chart which will be taken to the bank were credit will be applied for.

Designated employees – cook cleaner chef, these staff will be hired and put on a contract totaling a sum of 60.000 pounds on commission for the annum five chefs two cleaners and a head chef.

Refurbishments furnishings – floor boards toilets carpets sides and sinks will be the topic of refurbishments these will go on the cash flow chart for purchase, a carpet in the main diner floorboards in the upstairs Jacuzzi area toilets built and fitted with hygiene systems and kitchen sinks for different forms of washing.

Objective statement:

Business profile

Employees – nine staff will be employed each paid an annum salary of 20.000 pounds a year, they will sign a contract and a company policies contract stating all of the things needed of them to qualify for their position.

They will be given hours for their duty and expected to make good use of them.

A head chef will be hired for recipes and menus five cooks will be hired to accompany him and too cleaners for routine cleaning duties they will also manage and occupy the gymnasium area.

Routines – the head chef will be expected to arrive an hour early for work she will be expected to open up shop, order produce for cooking and supplying food, instruct the kitchen on how to use utensils and make decent food from original recipes.

Cooks arrive early for work listen to what the head chef is telling them to do cook and prepare meals to a clean and hygienic order, keep the kitchen area clean and sanitized continually washing hands whilst serving up dishes.

Cleaners will be expected to arrive early for work take up their products, wear a cleaning goon and attend to cleaning duties they will also be in charge of the management of the Jacuzzi area, taking appointments and nursing customers.

Duties – head chef supply recipes managing the kitchen keeping health and safety in order, stocking cabinets pulling groceries maintaining the hygiene of the cooks. Cleaning the building regularly maintaining the health and safety of building, taking appointments of clients for spa treatment.

Title – restaurant

Advantages – this restaurant will have better cooks with a more decent serving etiquette then any other restaurant in the area, the catering will be managed responsibly and to a decent standard.

Health and safety – this will be written out on the rules and regulations and go down on the wall of the kitchen diner it will be attached to the contract along with the company policies statement sheet and be signed by the employee candidate.

Company policies –

Supplies -

Business aim:

2-3-7

Cash flow chart
Cost
Property

Renovations
Refurbishments
Furnishings
Total

The cost of the property will be roughly 200 grand
The renovation of the property will be roughly ten thousand
For refurbishment the cost estimates 5k
The furnishings will come too around 20.000

A spacious building pine floorboard newly fitted hygienic toilets carpets a kitchen side ten sinks, a Jacuzzi a refrigerator ten cookers four ovens a well fitted kitchen with a full apparatus.

Administration – monies will be handled with responsibility and profession.

Management – the administrator will handled the percentage and shares of finance

Organization – paperwork reports and contracts will be negotiated to ledger signature

Supervision – credit will be observed frequently to ensure continuity is honest

Regulation – contracts will be followed and pursued for business aims intent

Instruction – paperwork and finance advance permission forms will be available

Finance – money will be put too good use economy investments will be valid

Administration fees
Fees -
Bills -
Debts -
Loans –
Costs -
Arrangements –

Contract Financial arrangements:
Premium bond
Profits
Annum gross
Merchandise subsidiary
Project statement

References – local businesses associated with area of clinic management could be used as a reference for the supply of grocery. (Local tesco manager)

Equities – get a base rate loan from the bank of around 500.000 then pay them back on a five-year repayment scheme.

Produce – the possibility of a farm in the near future where cattle are herded, crops are grown.

Groceries – will be supplied by the local supermarket and looked for in and around the town.

Legislation - a solicitor and a police officer will be called in to sign any contracts with the bank that need looking at. They can also become senior partners in the health clinic industry.

Contracts – three page distinctive contracts will be written for the staff and duty management of employees, these contracts will state company policies their rate of pay opening times shifts holidays work periods contact and registration details illness's and any special needs that they might have.

Registration - get the business registered at HM and revenue or at a regional tax office.

Certification – get the business certified at HM and revenue or at a regional tax office.

www.ingramcontent.com/pod-product-compliance
Lightning Source LLC
Chambersburg PA
CBHW021046180526
45163CB00005B/2307